SIMPLY KETO WORKBOOK

by

Susan Ryan

LIVE

LOVE

KETO

Track Your Progress

Day .... Date.................

- **Diet Plan**

  ....
  ....
  ....

- **How do you feel?**

  ....
  ....
  ....
  ....

- **Record your weight:** ....

<u>Track Your Progress</u>

Day ....   **Date**.................

- ## <u>Diet Plan</u>

> ....
>
> ....

- ## <u>How do you feel?</u>

> ....
>
> ....
>
> ....

- ## Record your weight: ....

Track Your Progress

Day ....   **Date**.................

- ## Diet Plan

....
....
....

- ## How do you feel?

....
....
....
....

- ## Record your weight: ....

<u>Track Your Progress</u>

Day ....   **Date**..................

- ### <u>Diet Plan</u>

....

....

- ### <u>How do you feel?</u>

....

....

....

- ### Record your weight: ....

Track Your Progress

Day ....   **Date**.................

- ## Diet Plan

....
....
....

- ## How do you feel?

....
....
....
....

- ## Record your weight: ....

<u>Track Your Progress</u>

Day ....   **Date**.................

- ## <u>Diet Plan</u>

....

....

- ## <u>How do you feel?</u>

....

....

....

- ## Record your weight: ....

Track Your Progress

Day .... Date.................

- **Diet Plan**

....

....

....

- **How do you feel?**

....

....

....

....

- **Record your weight: ....**

Track Your Progress

Day ....   Date..................

- **Diet Plan**

  ....

  ....

- **How do you feel?**

  ....

  ....

  ....

- **Record your weight: ....**

KETO WORKBOOK
LIVE **&** LOVE **KETO**

Track Your Progress

Day .... **Date**.................

- ### Diet Plan

  ....
  ....
  ....

- ### How do you feel?

  ....
  ....
  ....
  ....

- **Record your weight:** ....

Track Your Progress

Day ....   **Date**.................

- ### Diet Plan

> ....
>
> ....

- ### How do you feel?

> ....
>
> ....
>
> ....

- ### Record your weight: ....

Track Your Progress

Day ....   **Date**..................

- ### Diet Plan

....
....

- ### How do you feel?

....
....
....

- ### Record your weight: ....

Track Your Progress

Day .... Date.................

- **<u>Diet Plan</u>**

  ....
  ....
  ....

- **<u>How do you feel?</u>**

  ....
  ....
  ....
  ....

- **Record your weight: ....**

Track Your Progress

Day ....   **Date**..................

- ## Diet Plan

> ....
>
> ....

- ## How do you feel?

> ....
>
> ....
>
> ....

- ## Record your weight: ....

Track Your Progress

Day ....   **Date**..................

- ## Diet Plan

  ....
  ....
  ....

- ## How do you feel?

  ....
  ....
  ....
  ....

- **Record your weight:** ....

KETO WORKBOOK

LIVE & LOVE KETO

<u>Track Your Progress</u>

Day ....   **Date**.................

- ## <u>Diet Plan</u>

> ....
>
> ....
....

- ## <u>How do you feel?</u>

> ....
>
> ....
>
> ....
....

- ## Record your weight: ....

Track Your Progress

Day ....   **Date**.................

- ## Diet Plan

> ....
>
> ....

- ## How do you feel?

> ....
>
> ....
>
> ....

- **Record your weight:** ....

Track Your Progress

Day ....   **Date**.................

- ## Diet Plan

- ## How do you feel?

- ## Record your weight: ....

Track Your Progress

Day ....   **Date**..................

- ## Diet Plan

  ....

  ....

- ## How do you feel?

  ....

  ....

  ....

- ## Record your weight: ....

KETO WORKBOOK
LIVE **&** LOVE **KETO**

Track Your Progress

Day ....   **Date**..................

- ## Diet Plan

  ....
  ....

- ## How do you feel?

  ....
  ....
  ....

- ## Record your weight: ....

Track Your Progress

Day ....   **Date**..................

- **Diet Plan**

- **How do you feel?**

- **Record your weight:** ....

Track Your Progress

Day ....   **Date**.................

- **Diet Plan**

- **How do you feel?**

- **Record your weight:** ....

Track Your Progress

Day ....   **Date**.................

- ## Diet Plan

  ....
  ....

- ## How do you feel?

  ....
  ....
  ....

- **Record your weight:** ....

Track Your Progress

Day .... **Date**.................

- **Diet Plan**

  ....
  ....
  ....

- **How do you feel?**

  ....
  ....
  ....
  ....

- **Record your weight:** ....

Track Your Progress

Day ....   **Date**..................

- ## Diet Plan

  ....
  ....
  ....

- ## How do you feel?

  ....
  ....
  ....
  ....

- ## Record your weight: ....

KETO WORKBOOK
LIVE **& LOVE KETO**

Track Your Progress

Day ....   Date..................

- **Diet Plan**

....

....

- **How do you feel?**

....

....

....

- **Record your weight:** ....

Track Your Progress

Day ....   **Date**..................

- ## Diet Plan

....
....

- ## How do you feel?

....
....
....

- ## Record your weight: ....

Track Your Progress

Day ....   Date.................

- ### Diet Plan

  ....
  ....

- ### How do you feel?

  ....
  ....
  ....

- ### Record your weight: ....

LIVE

LOVE

KETO

<u>Track Your Progress</u>

Day ....   **Date**..................

- ## <u>Diet Plan</u>

....

....

- ## <u>How do you feel?</u>

....

....

....

- ## Record your weight: ....

Track Your Progress

Day ....   Date..................

- ### Diet Plan

  ....
  ....
  ....

- ### How do you feel?

  ....
  ....
  ....
  ....

- ### Record your weight: ....

Track Your Progress

Day .... Date.................

- **Diet Plan**

  ....
  ....
  ....

- **How do you feel?**

  ....
  ....
  ....
  ....

- **Record your weight:** ....

<u>Track Your Progress</u>

Day ....   **Date**.................

- ## <u>Diet Plan</u>

....
....

- ## <u>How do you feel?</u>

....
....
....

- ## Record your weight: ....

Track Your Progress

Day .... **Date**.................

- ### Diet Plan

....
....

- ### How do you feel?

....
....
....

- ### Record your weight: ....

Track Your Progress

Day ....   **Date**.................

- ## Diet Plan

....
....

- ## How do you feel?

....
....
....

- **Record your weight:** ....

Track Your Progress

Day ....   Date..................

- **<u>Diet Plan</u>**

  ....
  ....

- **<u>How do you feel?</u>**

  ....
  ....
  ....

- **Record your weight: ....**

Track Your Progress

Day .... **Date**..................

- **Diet Plan**

- **How do you feel?**

- **Record your weight:** ....

Track Your Progress

Day .... **Date**.................

- ### Diet Plan

  ....
  ....
  ....

- ### How do you feel?

  ....
  ....
  ....
  ....

- ### Record your weight: ....

Track Your Progress

Day ....   **Date**.................

- ### Diet Plan

....
....

- ### How do you feel?

....
....
....

- ### Record your weight: ....

Track Your Progress

Day ....   **Date**.................

- ## Diet Plan

  ....
  ....
  ....

- ## How do you feel?

  ....
  ....
  ....
  ....

- ## Record your weight: ....

Track Your Progress

Day ....   **Date**.................

- ## Diet Plan

....
....

- ## How do you feel?

....
....
....

- **Record your weight:** ....

<u>Track Your Progress</u>

Day .... **Date**..................

- ### <u>Diet Plan</u>

> ....
> ....
> ....

- ### <u>How do you feel?</u>

> ....
> ....
> ....
> ....

- ### Record your weight: ....

Track Your Progress

Day ....   **Date**.................

- **Diet Plan**

- **How do you feel?**

- **Record your weight:** ....

Track Your Progress

Day .... Date.................

- **Diet Plan**

- **How do you feel?**

- **Record your weight:** ....

Track Your Progress

Day ....   Date.................

- ## Diet Plan

  ....
  ....

- ## How do you feel?

  ....
  ....
  ....

- ## Record your weight: ....

Track Your Progress

Day ....   **Date**.................

- ### Diet Plan

....
....

- ### How do you feel?

....
....
....

- ### Record your weight: ....

Track Your Progress

Day ....   **Date**.................

- ## **Diet Plan**

....

....

....

- ## **How do you feel?**

....

....

....

....

- ## **Record your weight:** ....

Track Your Progress

Day ....   **Date**..................

- ### Diet Plan

....
....

- ### How do you feel?

....
....
....

- **Record your weight:** ....

Track Your Progress

Day ....   Date.................

- ### Diet Plan

....
....

- ### How do you feel?

....
....
....

- **Record your weight: ....**

Track Your Progress

Day .... **Date**.................

- ### Diet Plan

  ....
  ....
  ....

- ### How do you feel?

  ....
  ....
  ....
  ....

- ### Record your weight: ....

<u>Track Your Progress</u>

Day ………………….   **Date**…………….

- ## <u>Diet Plan</u>

  ……………………………………………………………………………
  ……………………………………………………………………………

- ## <u>How do you feel?</u>

  ……………………………………………………………………………
  ……………………………………………………………………………
  ……………………………………………………………………………

- ## Record your weight: ……………………

<u>Track Your Progress</u>

Day ....   **Date**..................

- ## <u>Diet Plan</u>

....
....

- ## <u>How do you feel?</u>

....
....
....

- ## Record your weight: ....

Track Your Progress

Day .... **Date**.................

- **Diet Plan**

- **How do you feel?**

- **Record your weight:** ....

Track Your Progress

Day .... **Date**..................

- **Diet Plan**

....
....

- **How do you feel?**

....
....
....

- **Record your weight:** ....

<u>Track Your Progress</u>

Day ....   **Date**.................

- ## <u>Diet Plan</u>

  ....

  ....

- ## <u>How do you feel?</u>

  ....

  ....

  ....

- ## Record your weight: ....

Track Your Progress

Day ....   **Date**.................

- ## Diet Plan

  ....
  ....
  ....

- ## How do you feel?

  ....
  ....
  ....
  ....

- ## Record your weight: ....

Track Your Progress

Day .... Date.................

- ## Diet Plan

....
....
....

- ## How do you feel?

....
....
....
....

- **Record your weight: ....**

LIVE

LOVE

KETO

Track Your Progress

Day .... **Date**................

- ## Diet Plan

  ....
  ....
  ....

- ## How do you feel?

  ....
  ....
  ....
  ....

- ## Record your weight: ....

Track Your Progress

Day ……………………   **Date**……………….

- ## Diet Plan

  …………………………………………………………………………………………
  …………………………………………………………………………………………

- ## How do you feel?

  …………………………………………………………………………………………
  …………………………………………………………………………………………
  …………………………………………………………………………………………

- ## Record your weight: ……………………

<u>Track Your Progress</u>

Day ....   **Date**..................

- ## <u>Diet Plan</u>

> ....
>
> ....
>
> ....

- ## <u>How do you feel?</u>

> ....
>
> ....
>
> ....
>
> ....

- ## Record your weight: ....

Track Your Progress

Day ....   **Date**.................

- ## Diet Plan

> ....
>
> ....

- ## How do you feel?

> ....
>
> ....
>
> ....

- ## Record your weight: ....

Track Your Progress

Day ....   **Date**.................

- ## Diet Plan

> ....
>
> ....

- ## How do you feel?

> ....
>
> ....
>
> ....

- ## Record your weight: ....

Track Your Progress

Day .... **Date**................

- **Diet Plan**

  ....
  ....
  ....

- **How do you feel?**

  ....
  ....
  ....
  ....

- **Record your weight:** ....

Track Your Progress

Day .... Date.................

- ### Diet Plan

....
....

- ### How do you feel?

....
....
....

- **Record your weight: ....**

Track Your Progress

Day ....   **Date**..................

- ## Diet Plan

....

....

....

- ## How do you feel?

....

....

....

....

- **Record your weight:** ....

Track Your Progress

Day ....   **Date**.................

- ## Diet Plan

  ....
  ....
  ....

- ## How do you feel?

  ....
  ....
  ....
  ....

- ## Record your weight: ....

Track Your Progress

Day ....   **Date**.................

- **Diet Plan**

  ....

  ....

  ....

- **How do you feel?**

  ....

  ....

  ....

  ....

- **Record your weight:** ....

Track Your Progress

Day .... **Date**..................

- **Diet Plan**

- **How do you feel?**

- **Record your weight:** ....

<u>Track Your Progress</u>

Day .... **Date**.................

- ### <u>Diet Plan</u>

> ....
>
> ....

- ### <u>How do you feel?</u>

> ....
>
> ....
>
> ....

- ### Record your weight: ....

Track Your Progress

Day ....   **Date**.................

- **Diet Plan**

....
....

- **How do you feel?**

....
....
....

- **Record your weight: ....**

Track Your Progress

Day ....   **Date**..................

- **Diet Plan**

  ....

  ....

- **How do you feel?**

  ....

  ....

  ....

- **Record your weight: ....**

<u>Track Your Progress</u>

Day ....   **Date**..................

- ### <u>Diet Plan</u>

> ....
>
> ....

- ### <u>How do you feel?</u>

> ....
>
> ....
>
> ....

- ### Record your weight: ....

Track Your Progress

Day ....   **Date**..................

- **Diet Plan**

- **How do you feel?**

- **Record your weight:** ....

Track Your Progress

Day ....   **Date**................

- ## Diet Plan

  ....
  ....

- ## How do you feel?

  ....
  ....
  ....

- ## Record your weight: ....

Track Your Progress

Day ....   **Date**.................

- ## Diet Plan

  ....
  ....

- ## How do you feel?

  ....
  ....
  ....

- ## Record your weight: ....

Track Your Progress

Day ....   **Date**.................

- ## Diet Plan

....
....
....

- ## How do you feel?

....
....
....
....

- ## Record your weight: ....

Track Your Progress

Day .... **Date**..................

- **Diet Plan**

- **How do you feel?**

- **Record your weight:** ....

Track Your Progress

Day ....   **Date**..................

- ## Diet Plan

  ....

  ....

- ## How do you feel?

  ....

  ....

  ....

- **Record your weight:** ....

Track Your Progress

Day ....   **Date**..................

- ## Diet Plan

  ....
  ....
  ....

- ## How do you feel?

  ....
  ....
  ....
  ....

- ## Record your weight: ....

Track Your Progress

Day ....   **Date**.................

- ## Diet Plan

  ....
  ....

- ## How do you feel?

  ....
  ....
  ....

- **Record your weight:** ....

Track Your Progress

Day ....   Date..................

- ### Diet Plan

  ....
  ....
  ....

- ### How do you feel?

  ....
  ....
  ....
  ....

- ### Record your weight: ....

Track Your Progress

Day ....   **Date**..................

- ## Diet Plan

....
....

- ## How do you feel?

....
....
....

- ## Record your weight: ....

Track Your Progress

Day ....   **Date**..................

- ## Diet Plan

  ....
  ....

- ## How do you feel?

  ....
  ....
  ....

- ## Record your weight: ....

Track Your Progress

Day ....   **Date**..................

• **Diet Plan**

• **How do you feel?**

• **Record your weight:** ....

Track Your Progress

Day ....   **Date**..................

- ## Diet Plan

....
....

- ## How do you feel?

....
....
....

- ## Record your weight: ....

Track Your Progress

Day .... Date.................

- ## Diet Plan

....
....

- ## How do you feel?

....
....
....

- **Record your weight: ....**

LIVE

LOVE

KETO

Track Your Progress

Day ....   **Date**.................

- ## Diet Plan

....
....
....

- ## How do you feel?

....
....
....
....

- ## Record your weight: ....

Track Your Progress

Day ....   Date.................

- ## Diet Plan

....
....

- ## How do you feel?

....
....
....

- ## Record your weight: ....

Track Your Progress

Day ....   Date..................

- **Diet Plan**

  ....
  ....

- **How do you feel?**

  ....
  ....
  ....

- **Record your weight: ....**

Track Your Progress

Day ....   **Date**.................

- ## Diet Plan

  ....
  ....

- ## How do you feel?

  ....
  ....
  ....

- ## Record your weight: ....

<u>Track Your Progress</u>

Day ....   **Date**.................

- ## <u>Diet Plan</u>

> ....
>
> ....

- ## <u>How do you feel?</u>

> ....
>
> ....
>
> ....

- ## Record your weight: ....

Track Your Progress

Day ....   Date................

- ## Diet Plan

....
....

- ## How do you feel?

....
....
....

- ## Record your weight: ....

Track Your Progress

Day .... Date.................

• **Diet Plan**

....
....

• **How do you feel?**

....
....
....

• **Record your weight: ....**

KETO WORKBOOK
LIVE & LOVE KETO

Track Your Progress

Day .... **Date**.................

- ## Diet Plan

> ....
> ....

- ## How do you feel?

> ....
> ....
> ....

- **Record your weight:** ....

<u>Track Your Progress</u>

Day ....   **Date**.................

- ## <u>Diet Plan</u>

....
....

- ## <u>How do you feel?</u>

....
....
....

- ## Record your weight: ....

<u>Track Your Progress</u>

Day ....   **Date**.................

- ## <u>Diet Plan</u>

....
....

- ## <u>How do you feel?</u>

....
....
....

- ## Record your weight: ....

Track Your Progress

Day ....   **Date**.................

- ## Diet Plan

....
....

- ## How do you feel?

....
....
....

- **Record your weight:** ....

<u>Track Your Progress</u>

Day .... **Date**.................

- ### <u>Diet Plan</u>

....
....

- ### <u>How do you feel?</u>

....
....
....

- ### Record your weight: ....

Track Your Progress

Day ....   **Date**.................

- ## Diet Plan

  ....
  ....

- ## How do you feel?

  ....
  ....
  ....

- ## Record your weight: ....

Track Your Progress

Day ....   **Date**.................

- ## Diet Plan

  ....

  ....

- ## How do you feel?

  ....

  ....

  ....

- ## Record your weight: ....

Track Your Progress

Day .... **Date**.................

- **Diet Plan**

- **How do you feel?**

- **Record your weight:** ....

Track Your Progress

Day ....   **Date**..................

- ## Diet Plan

  ....

  ....

  ....

- ## How do you feel?

  ....

  ....

  ....

  ....

- ## Record your weight: ....

Track Your Progress

Day ....   **Date**.................

- ### Diet Plan

> ....
> ....

- ### How do you feel?

> ....
> ....
> ....

- ### Record your weight: ....

Track Your Progress

Day .... **Date**..................

- ### Diet Plan

  ....
  ....

- ### How do you feel?

  ....
  ....
  ....

- ### Record your weight: ....

Track Your Progress

Day ....   **Date**.................

- ## Diet Plan

  ....
  ....

- ## How do you feel?

  ....
  ....
  ....

- ## Record your weight: ....

Track Your Progress

Day ....   **Date**.................

- **Diet Plan**

- **How do you feel?**

- **Record your weight:** ....

Track Your Progress

Day .... Date..................

- **<u>Diet Plan</u>**

....
....

- **<u>How do you feel?</u>**

....
....
....

- **Record your weight: ....**

<u>Track Your Progress</u>

Day .... **Date**..................

- ## <u>Diet Plan</u>

> ....
>
> ....
>
> ....

- ## <u>How do you feel?</u>

> ....
>
> ....
>
> ....
>
> ....

- ## Record your weight: ....

Track Your Progress

Day ....   **Date**.................

- ## Diet Plan

  ....
  ....
  ....

- ## How do you feel?

  ....
  ....
  ....
  ....

- ## Record your weight: ....

KETO WORKBOOK

LIVE **& LOVE KETO**

Track Your Progress

Day ....   **Date**.................

- ## Diet Plan

  ....
  ....

- ## How do you feel?

  ....
  ....
  ....

- ## Record your weight: ....

<u>Track Your Progress</u>

Day ....   **Date**.................

- ## <u>Diet Plan</u>

  ....
  ....

- ## <u>How do you feel?</u>

  ....
  ....
  ....

- ## Record your weight: ....

Track Your Progress

Day ....   **Date**.................

- ## Diet Plan

....

....

- ## How do you feel?

....

....

....

- ## Record your weight: ....

Track Your Progress

Day ....   Date.................

- ## Diet Plan

....
....

- ## How do you feel?

....
....
....

- ## Record your weight: ....

Track Your Progress

Day .... **Date**.................

- **Diet Plan**

....
....

- **How do you feel?**

....
....
....

- **Record your weight:** ....

Track Your Progress

Day ....   **Date**..................

- **Diet Plan**

  ```
  ....................................................
  ....................................................
  ....................................................
  ```

- **How do you feel?**

  ```
  ....................................................
  ....................................................
  ....................................................
  ....................................................
  ```

- **Record your weight: ....**

Track Your Progress

Day ....   **Date**..................

- ### Diet Plan

  ....

  ....

- ### How do you feel?

  ....

  ....

  ....

- ### Record your weight: ....

LIVE

LOVE

KETO

Track Your Progress

Day .... **Date**.................

- ## **Diet Plan**

- ## **How do you feel?**

- **Record your weight:** ....

Track Your Progress

Day ....   **Date**..................

- ## Diet Plan

....

....

....

- ## How do you feel?

....

....

....

....

- ## Record your weight: ....

Track Your Progress

Day .... **Date**..................

- **Diet Plan**

- **How do you feel?**

- **Record your weight:** ....

Track Your Progress

Day ....   **Date**.................

- ## Diet Plan

  ....
  ....

- ## How do you feel?

  ....
  ....
  ....

- ## Record your weight: ....

Track Your Progress

Day ....   Date.................

- ## Diet Plan

....

....

- ## How do you feel?

....

....

....

- ## Record your weight: ....

KETO WORKBOOK

LIVE **& LOVE KETO**

Track Your Progress

Day ....   **Date**.................

- ## Diet Plan

  ....
  ....

- ## How do you feel?

  ....
  ....
  ....

- ## Record your weight: ....

Track Your Progress

Day .... **Date**..................

- **Diet Plan**

- **How do you feel?**

- **Record your weight:** ....

Track Your Progress

Day ....   **Date**.................

- ## Diet Plan

  ....
  ....
  ....

- ## How do you feel?

  ....
  ....
  ....
  ....

- **Record your weight:** ....

Track Your Progress

Day ....   **Date**..................

- ## Diet Plan

  ....
  ....
  ....

- ## How do you feel?

  ....
  ....
  ....
  ....

- ## Record your weight: ....

Track Your Progress

Day ....   **Date**.................

- **Diet Plan**

  ....
  ....
  ....

- **How do you feel?**

  ....
  ....
  ....
  ....

- **Record your weight: ....**

Track Your Progress

Day .... **Date**.................

- ### Diet Plan

....
....

- ### How do you feel?

....
....
....

- ### Record your weight: ....

Track Your Progress

Day …………………….   **Date**………………..

- ## Diet Plan

  …………………………………………………………………
  …………………………………………………………………

- ## How do you feel?

  …………………………………………………………………
  …………………………………………………………………
  …………………………………………………………………

- ## Record your weight: …………………….

Track Your Progress

Day .... **Date**.................

- ## Diet Plan

....
....

- ## How do you feel?

....
....
....

- **Record your weight: ....**

Track Your Progress

Day ....   **Date**..................

- ## Diet Plan

  ....
  ....

- ## How do you feel?

  ....
  ....
  ....

- ## Record your weight: ....

Track Your Progress

Day ....   **Date**..................

- ### Diet Plan

  ....
  ....

- ### How do you feel?

  ....
  ....
  ....

- ### Record your weight: ....

Track Your Progress

Day ....   **Date**..................

- ## Diet Plan

....
....
....

- ## How do you feel?

....
....
....
....

- ## Record your weight: ....

Track Your Progress

Day ....   **Date**.................

- ## Diet Plan

  ....
  ....

- ## How do you feel?

  ....
  ....
  ....

- **Record your weight:** ....

Track Your Progress

Day .... **Date**..................

- ## Diet Plan

....

....

....

- ## How do you feel?

....

....

....

- ## Record your weight: ....

KETO WORKBOOK
LIVE **&** LOVE **KETO**

Track Your Progress

Day ....   **Date**.................

- **Diet Plan**

....

....

- **How do you feel?**

....

....

....

- **Record your weight:** ....

Track Your Progress

Day ....   **Date**.................

- ## Diet Plan

  ....
  ....
  ....

- ## How do you feel?

  ....
  ....
  ....
  ....

- ## Record your weight: ....

Track Your Progress

Day .... **Date**..................

- ### Diet Plan

  ....
  ....
  ....

- ### How do you feel?

  ....
  ....
  ....
  ....

- ### Record your weight: ....

<u>Track Your Progress</u>

Day ....   **Date**................,....

- ## <u>Diet Plan</u>

  ....
  ....

- ## <u>How do you feel?</u>

  ....
  ....
  ....

- ## Record your weight: ....

Track Your Progress

Day ....   **Date**.................

- ## Diet Plan

  ....
  ....

- ## How do you feel?

  ....
  ....
  ....

- ## Record your weight: ....

Track Your Progress

Day .... **Date**..................

- ## Diet Plan

> ....
>
> ....

- ## How do you feel?

> ....
>
> ....
>
> ....

- ## Record your weight: ....

Track Your Progress

Day ....   **Date**.................

- ## Diet Plan

  ....
  ....

- ## How do you feel?

  ....
  ....
  ....

- ## Record your weight: ....

Track Your Progress

Day ....   Date.................

- **Diet Plan**

  ....
  ....
  ....

- **How do you feel?**

  ....
  ....
  ....
  ....

- **Record your weight: ....**

Track Your Progress

Day .... Date.................

- ## Diet Plan

  ....
  ....
  ....

- ## How do you feel?

  ....
  ....
  ....
  ....

- ## Record your weight: ....

Track Your Progress

Day ....   **Date**.................

- ## Diet Plan

....
....

- ## How do you feel?

....
....
....

- **Record your weight:** ....

LIVE

LOVE

KETO

Track Your Progress

Day ....   **Date**..................

- ### Diet Plan

  ```
  ..............................................................
  ..............................................................
  ..............................................................
  ```

- ### How do you feel?

  ```
  ..............................................................
  ..............................................................
  ..............................................................
  ..............................................................
  ```

- ### Record your weight: ....

Track Your Progress

Day ....   **Date**.................

- ### Diet Plan

- ### How do you feel?

- ### Record your weight: ....

Track Your Progress

Day .... Date..................

- ## Diet Plan

> ....
>
> ....

- ## How do you feel?

> ....
>
> ....
>
> ....

- ## Record your weight: ....

Track Your Progress

Day ....   **Date**..................

- ## Diet Plan

  ....
  ....
  ....

- ## How do you feel?

  ....
  ....
  ....
  ....

- ## Record your weight: ....

Track Your Progress

Day .... Date.................

- ## Diet Plan

....
....

- ## How do you feel?

....
....
....

- **Record your weight: ....**

Track Your Progress

Day .... Date.................

- **<u>Diet Plan</u>**

  ....
  ....

- **<u>How do you feel?</u>**

  ....
  ....
  ....

- **Record your weight: ....**

Track Your Progress

Day ………………….   **Date**……………….

- ## Diet Plan

  ....
  ....

- ## How do you feel?

  ....
  ....
  ....

- ## Record your weight: …………………….

Track Your Progress

Day ....   **Date** ....

- **Diet Plan**

....
....

- **How do you feel?**

....
....
....

- **Record your weight:** ....

Track Your Progress

Day ....   **Date**.................

- ### Diet Plan

  ....
  ....

- ### How do you feel?

  ....
  ....
  ....

- ### Record your weight: ....

Track Your Progress

Day ....   **Date**.................

- ## Diet Plan

....
....
....

- ## How do you feel?

....
....
....

- ## Record your weight: ....

Track Your Progress

Day ....   **Date**..................

- ## Diet Plan

> ....
> ....
> ....

- ## How do you feel?

> ....
> ....
> ....
> ....

- ## Record your weight: ....

Track Your Progress

Day .... Date.................

- ## Diet Plan

....
....

- ## How do you feel?

....
....
....

- **Record your weight: ....**

Track Your Progress

Day .... **Date**..................

- ## Diet Plan

  ....

  ....

- ## How do you feel?

  ....

  ....

  ....

- ## Record your weight: ....

Track Your Progress

Day ....   **Date**.................

- **Diet Plan**

  ....
  ....

- **How do you feel?**

  ....
  ....
  ....

- **Record your weight:** ....

Track Your Progress

Day ....   Date..................

- **Diet Plan**

  ....
  ....
  ....

- **How do you feel?**

  ....
  ....
  ....
  ....

- **Record your weight: ....**

Track Your Progress

Day ....   **Date**.................

- ## Diet Plan

....

....

- ## How do you feel?

....

....

....

- ## Record your weight: ....

Track Your Progress

Day ....   **Date**.................

- ## Diet Plan

....

....

- ## How do you feel?

....

....

....

- ## Record your weight: ....

Track Your Progress

Day ....   Date.................

- ## Diet Plan

  ....
  ....

- ## How do you feel?

  ....
  ....
  ....

- ## Record your weight: ....

Track Your Progress

Day .... **Date**.................

- ## **Diet Plan**

....
....

- ## **How do you feel?**

....
....
....

- ## **Record your weight:** ....

Track Your Progress

Day .... **Date** ....

- **Diet Plan**

- **How do you feel?**

- **Record your weight:** ....

Track Your Progress

Day ....   Date.................

- ### Diet Plan

....
....

- ### How do you feel?

....
....
....

- ### Record your weight: ....

Track Your Progress

Day ....   Date.................

- **Diet Plan**

  ....

  ....

- **How do you feel?**

  ....

  ....

  ....

- **Record your weight:** ....

Track Your Progress

Day .... **Date**.................

- ## Diet Plan

  ....
  ....

- ## How do you feel?

  ....
  ....
  ....

- ## Record your weight: ....

Track Your Progress

Day ....   Date..................

- ## Diet Plan

....

....

- ## How do you feel?

....

....

....

- ## Record your weight: ....

Track Your Progress

Day ....   **Date**.................

- ### Diet Plan

....
....
....

- ### How do you feel?

....
....
....
....

- ### Record your weight: ....

Track Your Progress

Day ....   **Date**.................

- ## Diet Plan

  ....
  ....

- ## How do you feel?

  ....
  ....
  ....

- **Record your weight:** ....

<u>Track Your Progress</u>

Day ....   **Date**.................

- **<u>Diet Plan</u>**

> ....
> ....
> ....

- **<u>How do you feel?</u>**

> ....
> ....
> ....
> ....

- **Record your weight: ....**

Track Your Progress

Day ....   **Date**..................

- ### Diet Plan

> ....
> ....
> ....

- ### How do you feel?

> ....
> ....
> ....
> ....

- ### Record your weight: ....

Track Your Progress

Day ....   **Date**..................

- ## Diet Plan

  ....
  ....

- ## How do you feel?

  ....
  ....
  ....

- ## Record your weight: ....

Track Your Progress

Day ....   **Date**.................

- ## Diet Plan

....
....

- ## How do you feel?

....
....
....

- **Record your weight:** ....

Track Your Progress

Day .... Date.................

- ## Diet Plan

  ....
  ....

- ## How do you feel?

  ....
  ....
  ....

- ## Record your weight: ....

Track Your Progress

Day .... **Date**..................

- ## Diet Plan

....
....

- ## How do you feel?

....
....
....

- ## Record your weight: ....

Track Your Progress

Day ....   Date..................

- ## Diet Plan

....
....

- ## How do you feel?

....
....
....

- ## Record your weight: ....

Track Your Progress

Day .... **Date**................

- ### Diet Plan

  ....
  ....

- ### How do you feel?

  ....
  ....
  ....

- **Record your weight:** ....

KETO WORKBOOK
LIVE **&** LOVE **KETO**

Track Your Progress

Day ....   **Date**..................

- ## Diet Plan

....
....

- ## How do you feel?

....
....
....

- **Record your weight:** ....

KETO WORKBOOK
LIVE & LOVE KETO

LIVE

LOVE

KETO

Track Your Progress

Day .... **Date**..................

- ## Diet Plan

  ....
  ....

- ## How do you feel?

  ....
  ....
  ....

- **Record your weight:** ....

Track Your Progress

Day ....   **Date**..................

- ## Diet Plan

....
....

- ## How do you feel?

....
....
....

- ## Record your weight: ....

Track Your Progress

Day ....   **Date**.................

- **Diet Plan**

- **How do you feel?**

- **Record your weight:** ....

Track Your Progress

Day ....   **Date**..................

- ### Diet Plan

  ....

  ....

- ### How do you feel?

  ....

  ....

  ....

- ### Record your weight: ....

Track Your Progress

Day .... **Date**.................

- **<u>Diet Plan</u>**

....
....

- **<u>How do you feel?</u>**

....
....
....

- **Record your weight:** ....

Track Your Progress

Day ....   **Date**..................

- ## Diet Plan

....

....

- ## How do you feel?

....

....

....

- ## Record your weight: ....

Track Your Progress

Day ....   **Date**.................

- ## Diet Plan

  ....
  ....

- ## How do you feel?

  ....
  ....
  ....

- ## Record your weight: ....

<u>Track Your Progress</u>

Day ....   **Date**.................

- ### <u>Diet Plan</u>

  ....
  ....

- ### <u>How do you feel?</u>

  ....
  ....
  ....

- ### Record your weight: ....

Track Your Progress

Day ....   **Date**..................

- ## Diet Plan

....
....
....

- ## How do you feel?

....
....
....
....

- ## Record your weight: ....

Track Your Progress

Day ....   **Date**.................

- ### Diet Plan

....
....

- ### How do you feel?

....
....
....

- ### Record your weight: ....

Track Your Progress

Day ....   **Date**.................

- ## Diet Plan

....
....

- ## How do you feel?

....
....
....

- ## Record your weight: ....

Track Your Progress

Day ....   **Date**.................

- ## Diet Plan

....
....

- ## How do you feel?

....
....
....

- **Record your weight: ....**

Track Your Progress

Day ....   **Date**..................

- ## Diet Plan

  ....
  ....
  ....

- ## How do you feel?

  ....
  ....
  ....
  ....

- ## Record your weight: ....

Track Your Progress

Day ....   **Date**.................

- ### Diet Plan

- ### How do you feel?

- ### Record your weight: ....

KETO WORKBOOK

LIVE **&** LOVE **KETO**

Track Your Progress

Day ....   Date..................

- ### Diet Plan

- ### How do you feel?

- ### Record your weight: ....

Track Your Progress

Day .... **Date**..................

- ## Diet Plan

  ....

  ....

- ## How do you feel?

  ....

  ....

  ....

- ## Record your weight: ....

Track Your Progress

Day ....   Date..................

- **Diet Plan**

  ....
  ....

- **How do you feel?**

  ....
  ....
  ....

- **Record your weight: ....**

Track Your Progress

Day .... **Date**.................

- ## Diet Plan

....
....

- ## How do you feel?

....
....
....

- ## Record your weight: ....

Track Your Progress

Day .... **Date**..................

- **Diet Plan**

....
....
....

- **How do you feel?**

....
....
....
....

- **Record your weight:** ....

Track Your Progress

Day .... **Date**.................

- ## Diet Plan

....
....

- ## How do you feel?

....
....
....

- **Record your weight:** ....

Track Your Progress

Day ....   **Date**..................

- ## Diet Plan

  ....
  ....
  ....

- ## How do you feel?

  ....
  ....
  ....
  ....

- ## Record your weight: ....

Track Your Progress

Day .... Date.................

- ### Diet Plan

  ....
  ....

- ### How do you feel?

  ....
  ....
  ....

- ### Record your weight: ....

<u>Track Your Progress</u>

Day ....   **Date**..................

- ## <u>Diet Plan</u>

....
....

- ## <u>How do you feel?</u>

....
....
....

- ## Record your weight: ....

Track Your Progress

Day ....   **Date**.................

- ## Diet Plan

....
....

- ## How do you feel?

....
....
....

- **Record your weight:** ....

Track Your Progress

Day ....   **Date**.................

- ## Diet Plan

> ....
>
> ....

- ## How do you feel?

> ....
>
> ....
>
> ....

- ## Record your weight: ....

Track Your Progress

Day ....   **Date**.................

- **Diet Plan**

....

....

- **How do you feel?**

....

....

....

- **Record your weight:** ....

Track Your Progress

Day ....   **Date**.................

- **Diet Plan**

....
....

- **How do you feel?**

....
....
....

- **Record your weight:** ....

Track Your Progress

Day ....   **Date**.................

- ## Diet Plan

  ....

  ....

- ## How do you feel?

  ....

  ....

  ....

- ## Record your weight: ....

KETO WORKBOOK
LIVE **& LOVE KETO**

Track Your Progress

Day ....   **Date**.................

- ## Diet Plan

  ....
  ....
  ....

- ## How do you feel?

  ....
  ....
  ....
  ....

- **Record your weight:** ....

Track Your Progress

Day ....   **Date**.................

- ## Diet Plan

....
....

- ## How do you feel?

....
....
....

- ## Record your weight: ....

LIVE

LOVE

KETO

Track Your Progress

Day .... **Date**................

- ## Diet Plan

  ....
  ....

- ## How do you feel?

  ....
  ....
  ....

- ## Record your weight: ....

Track Your Progress

Day ....   **Date**.................

- ## Diet Plan

  ....
  ....
  ....

- ## How do you feel?

  ....
  ....
  ....
  ....

- ## Record your weight: ....

Track Your Progress

Day ………………….. **Date**……………….

- ## Diet Plan

  ……………………………………………………………………
  ……………………………………………………………………
  ……………………………………………………………………

- ## How do you feel?

  ……………………………………………………………………
  ……………………………………………………………………
  ……………………………………………………………………
  ……………………………………………………………………

- ## Record your weight: …………………….

Track Your Progress

Day .... **Date**..................

- ## Diet Plan

....
....

- ## How do you feel?

....
....
....

- **Record your weight:** ....

Track Your Progress

Day .... **Date**.................

- ### Diet Plan

....
....

- ### How do you feel?

....
....
....

- **Record your weight:** ....

Track Your Progress

Day .... **Date**.................

- ## Diet Plan

....
....
....

- ## How do you feel?

....
....
....
....

- ## Record your weight: ....

Track Your Progress

Day .... **Date**.................

- **Diet Plan**

  ....
  ....

- **How do you feel?**

  ....
  ....
  ....

- **Record your weight:** ....

Track Your Progress

Day ....   **Date**.................

- ## Diet Plan

....

....

....

- ## How do you feel?

....

....

....

....

- ## Record your weight: ....

Track Your Progress

Day ....   **Date**..................

- ## Diet Plan

  ....

  ....

- ## How do you feel?

  ....

  ....

  ....

- ## Record your weight: ....

Track Your Progress

Day ....   **Date**..................

- ## Diet Plan

....

....

- ## How do you feel?

....

....

....

- **Record your weight:** ....

Track Your Progress

Day .... Date................

- **<u>Diet Plan</u>**

....
....

- **<u>How do you feel?</u>**

....
....
....

- **Record your weight: ....**

Track Your Progress

Day .... **Date**..................

- ## Diet Plan

....
....

- ## How do you feel?

....
....
....

- ## Record your weight: ....

Track Your Progress

Day .... **Date**..................

- ## Diet Plan

  ....
  ....

- ## How do you feel?

  ....
  ....
  ....

- ## Record your weight: ....

Track Your Progress

Day ....   **Date**..................

- ## Diet Plan

  ....
  ....

- ## How do you feel?

  ....
  ....
  ....

- **Record your weight:** ....

<u>Track Your Progress</u>

Day ....   **Date**.................

- ## <u>Diet Plan</u>

  ....
  ....

- ## <u>How do you feel?</u>

  ....
  ....
  ....

- ## Record your weight: ....

Track Your Progress

Day ....   **Date**.................

- ## Diet Plan

....
....

- ## How do you feel?

....
....
....

- ## Record your weight: ....

Track Your Progress

Day .... **Date**.................

- ## Diet Plan

  ....

  ....

- ## How do you feel?

  ....

  ....

  ....

- ## Record your weight: ....

Track Your Progress

Day .... **Date**.................

- ## Diet Plan

> ....
>
> ....

- ## How do you feel?

> ....
>
> ....
>
> ....

- ## Record your weight: ....

Track Your Progress

Day .... Date.................

- **Diet Plan**

- **How do you feel?**

- **Record your weight:** ....

Track Your Progress

Day .... **Date**................

- **Diet Plan**

....
....
....

- **How do you feel?**

....
....
....
....

- **Record your weight:** ....

Track Your Progress

Day ....   **Date**..................

- ### Diet Plan

  ....

  ....

- ### How do you feel?

  ....

  ....

  ....

- ### Record your weight: ....

Track Your Progress

Day ....   **Date**.................

- ## Diet Plan

....
....

- ## How do you feel?

....
....
....

- **Record your weight:** ....

Track Your Progress

Day ....   **Date**.................

- ## Diet Plan

  ....
  ....

- ## How do you feel?

  ....
  ....
  ....

- ## Record your weight: ....

Track Your Progress

Day ....   **Date**..................

- ## Diet Plan

....
....

- ## How do you feel?

....
....
....

- ## Record your weight: ....

<u>Track Your Progress</u>

Day ....   **Date**.................

- ## <u>Diet Plan</u>

  ....
  ....

- ## <u>How do you feel?</u>

  ....
  ....
  ....

- ## Record your weight: ....

Track Your Progress

Day ....   Date..................

- **<u>Diet Plan</u>**

> ....
>
> ....
>
> ....

- **<u>How do you feel?</u>**

> ....
>
> ....
>
> ....
>
> ....

- **Record your weight: ....**

Track Your Progress

Day ....   **Date**.................

- ## Diet Plan

  ....
  ....

- ## How do you feel?

  ....
  ....
  ....

- ## Record your weight: ....

Track Your Progress

Day ....   **Date**.................

- ## **Diet Plan**

....
....

- ## **How do you feel?**

....
....
....

- ## **Record your weight:** ....

Track Your Progress

Day ....   Date.................

- ### Diet Plan

....
....

- ### How do you feel?

....
....
....

- ### Record your weight: ....

Track Your Progress

Day .... **Date**..................

- **Diet Plan**

  ....
  ....

- **How do you feel?**

  ....
  ....
  ....

- **Record your weight:** ....

Track Your Progress

Day ....   **Date**.................

- ## Diet Plan

....

....

- ## How do you feel?

....

....

....

- ## Record your weight: ....

KETO WORKBOOK

LIVE **& LOVE KETO**

Track Your Progress

Day ....   Date..................

- ## <u>Diet Plan</u>

....
....

- ## <u>How do you feel?</u>

....
....
....

- ## Record your weight: ....

Track Your Progress

Day ....   Date.................

- ## Diet Plan

  ....
  ....

- ## How do you feel?

  ....
  ....
  ....

- ## Record your weight: ....

Track Your Progress

Day ....   **Date**..................

- **Diet Plan**

- **How do you feel?**

- **Record your weight:** ....

Track Your Progress

Day ....   **Date**.................

- ### Diet Plan

  ....
  ....

- ### How do you feel?

  ....
  ....
  ....

- ## Record your weight: ....

Track Your Progress

Day .... Date..................

- ### Diet Plan

....
....

- ### How do you feel?

....
....
....

- ### Record your weight: ....

Track Your Progress

Day ....   **Date**................

- ## Diet Plan

....

....

- ## How do you feel?

....

....

....

- ## Record your weight: ....

KETO WORKBOOK
LIVE **&** LOVE **KETO**

Track Your Progress

Day ....   Date.................

- ### Diet Plan

  ....
  ....

- ### How do you feel?

  ....
  ....
  ....

- ### Record your weight: ....

Track Your Progress

Day ....   **Date**..................

- ## Diet Plan

> ....
>
> ....

- ## How do you feel?

> ....
>
> ....
>
> ....

- ## Record your weight: ....

Track Your Progress

Day ....   **Date**..................

- ## Diet Plan

  ....
  ....

- ## How do you feel?

  ....
  ....
  ....

- ## Record your weight: ....

Track Your Progress

Day ....   **Date**.................

- ## Diet Plan

....
....
....

- ## How do you feel?

....
....
....
....

- **Record your weight: ....**

Track Your Progress

Day .... **Date**..................

- ## **Diet Plan**

....
....

- ## **How do you feel?**

....
....
....

- **Record your weight:** ....

Track Your Progress

Day .... **Date**.................

- ## Diet Plan

....
....

- ## How do you feel?

....
....
....

- **Record your weight:** ....

Track Your Progress

Day ....   Date.................

- ## Diet Plan

  ....
  ....

- ## How do you feel?

  ....
  ....
  ....

- ## Record your weight: ....

<u>Track Your Progress</u>

Day .... **Date**.................

- ## <u>Diet Plan</u>

....
....

- ## <u>How do you feel?</u>

....
....
....

- ## Record your weight: ....

Track Your Progress

Day ....   **Date**.................

- ## Diet Plan

....
....

- ## How do you feel?

....
....
....

- **Record your weight:** ....

LIVE

LOVE

KETO

Track Your Progress

Day ....   **Date**.................

- **Diet Plan**

....
....

- **How do you feel?**

....
....
....

- **Record your weight:** ....

Track Your Progress

Day .... **Date**.................

- ## Diet Plan

....
....

- ## How do you feel?

....
....
....

- ## Record your weight: ....

Track Your Progress

Day .... 　　　Date.................

- ## Diet Plan

....
....
....

- ## How do you feel?

....
....
....
....

- ## Record your weight: ....

Track Your Progress

Day .... **Date**.................

- ## Diet Plan

  ....
  ....
  ....

- ## How do you feel?

  ....
  ....
  ....
  ....

- ## Record your weight: ....

Track Your Progress

Day ....   Date.................

- ## Diet Plan

  ....
  ....

- ## How do you feel?

  ....
  ....
  ....

- **Record your weight: ....**

<u>Track Your Progress</u>

Day ....   **Date**.................

- ## <u>Diet Plan</u>

  ....
  ....

- ## <u>How do you feel?</u>

  ....
  ....
  ....

- ## Record your weight: ....

Track Your Progress

Day .... Date..................

- ## Diet Plan

  ....
  ....

- ## How do you feel?

  ....
  ....
  ....

- ## Record your weight: ....

Track Your Progress

Day .... Date.................

- **Diet Plan**

....
....

- **How do you feel?**

....
....
....

- **Record your weight:** ....

Track Your Progress

Day ....   **Date**..................

- ## Diet Plan

....
....
....

- ## How do you feel?

....
....
....
....

- ## Record your weight: ....

Track Your Progress

Day ....   Date..................

- ## Diet Plan

  ....
  ....

- ## How do you feel?

  ....
  ....
  ....

- ## Record your weight: ....

Track Your Progress

Day ....   **Date**.................

- ## Diet Plan

  ....
  ....

- ## How do you feel?

  ....
  ....
  ....

- **Record your weight: ....**

Track Your Progress

Day ....   Date.................

- ## Diet Plan

  ....
  ....
  ....

- ## How do you feel?

  ....
  ....
  ....
  ....

- ## Record your weight: ....

Track Your Progress

Day ....   **Date**................

- ## Diet Plan

....
....

- ## How do you feel?

....
....
....

- ## Record your weight: ....

Track Your Progress

Day .... **Date**.................

- ## **Diet Plan**

....
....

- ## **How do you feel?**

....
....
....

- ## **Record your weight:** ....

Track Your Progress

Day ....   **Date**.................

- ## Diet Plan

....
....

- ## How do you feel?

....
....
....

- **Record your weight:** ....

Track Your Progress

Day ....   **Date**..................

- **Diet Plan**

  ....
  ....

- **How do you feel?**

  ....
  ....
  ....

- **Record your weight:** ....

Track Your Progress

Day .... **Date**.................

- ## Diet Plan

....
....

- ## How do you feel?

....
....
....

- ## Record your weight: ....

Track Your Progress

Day .... **Date**.................

- ### Diet Plan

....
....

- ### How do you feel?

....
....
....

- **Record your weight:** ....

Track Your Progress

Day ....   **Date**................

- ## Diet Plan

....
....

- ## How do you feel?

....
....
....

- **Record your weight:** ....

Track Your Progress

Day .... **Date**.................

- ## Diet Plan

  ....
  ....

- ## How do you feel?

  ....
  ....
  ....

- ## Record your weight: ....

Track Your Progress

Day ....   **Date**.................

- ## Diet Plan

....
....

- ## How do you feel?

....
....
....

- **Record your weight: ....**

Track Your Progress

Day ....   Date.................

- ### Diet Plan

  ....
  ....
  ....

- ### How do you feel?

  ....
  ....
  ....
  ....

- **Record your weight: ....**

Track Your Progress

Day ....   **Date**..................

- ## <u>Diet Plan</u>

....

....

- ## <u>How do you feel?</u>

....

....

....

- ## Record your weight: ....

Track Your Progress

Day ....   Date.................

- ## Diet Plan

....
....
....

- ## How do you feel?

....
....
....
....

- **Record your weight: ....**

<u>Track Your Progress</u>

Day .... **Date**.................

- ## <u>Diet Plan</u>

....
....

- ## <u>How do you feel?</u>

....
....
....

- ## Record your weight: ....

Track Your Progress

Day ....   **Date**................

- ## Diet Plan

  ....
  ....

- ## How do you feel?

  ....
  ....
  ....

- ## Record your weight: ....

Track Your Progress

Day ....   **Date**..................

- ## Diet Plan

....
....

- ## How do you feel?

....
....
....

- ## Record your weight: ....

Track Your Progress

Day ....   **Date**...................

- ## Diet Plan

  ....
  ....

- ## How do you feel?

  ....
  ....
  ....

- ## Record your weight: ....

Track Your Progress

Day ....   **Date**..................

- ## Diet Plan

....
....

- ## How do you feel?

....
....
....

- ## Record your weight: ....

Track Your Progress

Day .... **Date**.................

- **Diet Plan**

....
....

- **How do you feel?**

....
....
....

- **Record your weight:** ....

KETO WORKBOOK
LIVE **& LOVE KETO**

Track Your Progress

Day .... Date.................

- ## Diet Plan

....
....

- ## How do you feel?

....
....
....

- ## Record your weight: ....

Track Your Progress

Day .... **Date**.................

- ## Diet Plan

  ....
  ....

- ## How do you feel?

  ....
  ....
  ....

- ## Record your weight: ....

LIVE

LOVE

KETO

Track Your Progress

Day ....   **Date**.................

- ## Diet Plan

....
....

- ## How do you feel?

....
....
....

- **Record your weight: ....**

<u>Track Your Progress</u>

Day ....   **Date**..................

- ## <u>Diet Plan</u>

....

....

....

- ## <u>How do you feel?</u>

....

....

....

....

- ## Record your weight: ....

Track Your Progress

Day .... **Date**.................

- ## Diet Plan

....
....

- ## How do you feel?

....
....
....

- **Record your weight:** ....

Track Your Progress

Day .... **Date**..................

- ## Diet Plan

....
....

- ## How do you feel?

....
....
....

- **Record your weight:** ....

Track Your Progress

Day ....   **Date**.................

- ## Diet Plan

  ....
  ....

- ## How do you feel?

  ....
  ....
  ....

- **Record your weight:** ....

Track Your Progress

Day ....   Date.................

- ## Diet Plan

....
....

- ## How do you feel?

....
....
....

- ## Record your weight: ....

Track Your Progress

Day ....   **Date**.................

- ### Diet Plan

....
....

- ### How do you feel?

....
....
....

- ## Record your weight: ....

Track Your Progress

Day .... Date.................

- ## Diet Plan

  ....
  ....

- ## How do you feel?

  ....
  ....
  ....

- **Record your weight: ....**

Track Your Progress

Day .... Date.................

- ## Diet Plan

- ## How do you feel?

- ## Record your weight: ....

Track Your Progress

Day ....   **Date**..................

- ## Diet Plan

....
....
....

- ## How do you feel?

....
....
....
....

- **Record your weight:** ....

Track Your Progress

Day .... Date..................

- ## Diet Plan

  ....
  ....

- ## How do you feel?

  ....
  ....
  ....

- ## Record your weight: ....

Track Your Progress

Day ....   Date.................

- ### Diet Plan

  ....
  ....

- ### How do you feel?

  ....
  ....
  ....

- ### Record your weight: ....

Track Your Progress

Day .... Date.................

- ## Diet Plan

....
....

- ## How do you feel?

....
....
....

- **Record your weight: ....**

Track Your Progress

Day ....   **Date**.................

- ## Diet Plan

....
....

- ## How do you feel?

....
....
....

- ## Record your weight: ....

Track Your Progress

Day .... **Date**.................

- ## Diet Plan

  ....
  ....

- ## How do you feel?

  ....
  ....
  ....

- ## Record your weight: ....

<u>Track Your Progress</u>

Day ....   **Date**.................

- ## <u>Diet Plan</u>

....
....

- ## <u>How do you feel?</u>

....
....
....

- ## Record your weight: ....

Track Your Progress

Day ....   **Date**.................

- ## Diet Plan

  ....
  ....

- ## How do you feel?

  ....
  ....
  ....

- **Record your weight:** ....

<u>Track Your Progress</u>

Day ....   **Date**.................

- ## <u>Diet Plan</u>

  ....
  ....

- ## <u>How do you feel?</u>

  ....
  ....
  ....

- ## Record your weight: ....

Track Your Progress

Day ....   **Date**.................

- ## Diet Plan

....

....

- ## How do you feel?

....

....

....

- ## Record your weight: ....

Track Your Progress

Day ....   **Date**..................

- ## Diet Plan

- ## How do you feel?

- ## Record your weight: ....

<u>Track Your Progress</u>

Day ....   Date.................

- ## <u>Diet Plan</u>

....
....

- ## <u>How do you feel?</u>

....
....
....

- ## Record your weight: ....

Track Your Progress

Day .... Date.................

- ## Diet Plan

....
....

- ## How do you feel?

....
....
....

- **Record your weight: ....**

Track Your Progress

Day .... **Date**.................

- ## Diet Plan

....
....

- ## How do you feel?

....
....
....

- ## Record your weight: ....

Track Your Progress

Day .... **Date**..................

- ## Diet Plan

  ....
  ....

- ## How do you feel?

  ....
  ....
  ....

- **Record your weight:** ....

Track Your Progress

Day .... Date.................

- ## Diet Plan

  ....
  ....

- ## How do you feel?

  ....
  ....
  ....

- ## Record your weight: ....

Track Your Progress

Day ....   Date..................

- ## **Diet Plan**

....
....
....

- ## **How do you feel?**

....
....
....
....

- ## **Record your weight:** ....

Track Your Progress

Day ....   **Date**.................

- ## Diet Plan

- ## How do you feel?

- ## Record your weight: ....

Track Your Progress

Day ....   **Date**..................

- ## Diet Plan

....
....

- ## How do you feel?

....
....
....

- ## Record your weight: ....

Track Your Progress

Day ....   **Date**.................

- ## Diet Plan

- ## How do you feel?

- ## Record your weight: ....

Track Your Progress

Day ....   Date.................

- ## Diet Plan

  ....
  ....

- ## How do you feel?

  ....
  ....
  ....

- ## Record your weight: ....

Track Your Progress

Day .... Date.................

- **Diet Plan**

....
....
....

- **How do you feel?**

....
....
....
....

- **Record your weight:** ....

Track Your Progress

Day ....   **Date**.................

- ## Diet Plan

....
....

- ## How do you feel?

....
....
....

- **Record your weight:** ....

Track Your Progress

Day .... Date.................

- ## Diet Plan

....
....

- ## How do you feel?

....
....
....

- **Record your weight:** ....

Track Your Progress

Day .... **Date**.................

- **Diet Plan**

- **How do you feel?**

- **Record your weight:** ....

Track Your Progress

Day ....   **Date**.................

- ## Diet Plan

  ....
  ....

- ## How do you feel?

  ....
  ....
  ....

- **Record your weight:** ....

Track Your Progress

Day ....   **Date**..................

- ## Diet Plan

  ....

  ....

- ## How do you feel?

  ....

  ....

  ....

- ## Record your weight: ....

Track Your Progress

Day .... **Date**.................

- ## Diet Plan

> ....
>
> ....

- ## How do you feel?

> ....
>
> ....
>
> ....

- **Record your weight:** ....

<u>Track Your Progress</u>

Day ....   **Date**..................

- ### <u>Diet Plan</u>

....
....

- ### <u>How do you feel?</u>

....
....
....

- ### Record your weight: ....

Track Your Progress

Day .... **Date**.................

- ## Diet Plan

  ....
  ....

- ## How do you feel?

  ....
  ....
  ....

- ## Record your weight: ....

<u>Track Your Progress</u>

Day .... **Date**..................

- ## <u>Diet Plan</u>

....
....

- ## <u>How do you feel?</u>

....
....
....

- ## Record your weight: ....

Track Your Progress

Day .... **Date**.................

- ## <u>Diet Plan</u>

....
....

- ## <u>How do you feel?</u>

....
....
....

- ## Record your weight: ....

LIVE

LOVE

KETO

Track Your Progress

Day ....   Date.................

- ## Diet Plan

  ....
  ....

- ## How do you feel?

  ....
  ....
  ....

- ## Record your weight: ....

Track Your Progress

Day ....   **Date**..................

- ## Diet Plan

....
....

- ## How do you feel?

....
....
....

- ## Record your weight: ....

Track Your Progress

Day ....   **Date**.................

- ## Diet Plan

- ## How do you feel?

- ## Record your weight: ....

Track Your Progress

Day ....   Date.................

- ## Diet Plan

> ....
>
> ....

- ## How do you feel?

> ....
>
> ....
>
> ....

- ## Record your weight: ....

Track Your Progress

Day ....   **Date**..................

- ### Diet Plan

  ....
  ....

- ### How do you feel?

  ....
  ....
  ....

- ### Record your weight: ....

Track Your Progress

Day ....   Date.................

- ## Diet Plan

  ....
  ....
  ....

- ## How do you feel?

  ....
  ....
  ....
  ....

- ## Record your weight: ....

Track Your Progress

Day .... Date.................

- ### Diet Plan

....
....

- ### How do you feel?

....
....
....

- ### Record your weight: ....

Track Your Progress

Day ....   Date.................

- ## Diet Plan

....
....

- ## How do you feel?

....
....
....

- **Record your weight:** ....

Track Your Progress

Day ....   Date.................

- ## Diet Plan

....
....
....

- ## How do you feel?

....
....
....
....

- ## Record your weight: ....

Track Your Progress

Day ....   **Date**.................

- ### Diet Plan

....
....

- ### How do you feel?

....
....
....

- ### Record your weight: ....

Track Your Progress

Day .... Date.................

• **<u>Diet Plan</u>**

....
....

• **<u>How do you feel?</u>**

....
....
....

• **Record your weight:** ....

Track Your Progress

Day ....   **Date**.................

- **Diet Plan**

  ....
  ....

- **How do you feel?**

  ....
  ....
  ....

- **Record your weight:** ....

Track Your Progress

Day ....   Date.................

- ## Diet Plan

  ....
  ....

- ## How do you feel?

  ....
  ....
  ....

- **Record your weight: ....**

<u>Track Your Progress</u>

Day ....   **Date**..................

- ## <u>Diet Plan</u>

....
....
....

- ## <u>How do you feel?</u>

....
....
....
....

- ## Record your weight: ....

Track Your Progress

Day ....   **Date**.................

- **Diet Plan**

  ....
  ....

- **How do you feel?**

  ....
  ....
  ....

- **Record your weight:** ....

Track Your Progress

Day .... **Date**.................

- ## Diet Plan

  ....
  ....

- ## How do you feel?

  ....
  ....
  ....

- ## Record your weight: ....

Track Your Progress

Day ....   Date................

- **Diet Plan**

  ....
  ....

- **How do you feel?**

  ....
  ....
  ....

- **Record your weight:** ....

Track Your Progress

Day ....   **Date**.................

- ## Diet Plan

  ....
  ....

- ## How do you feel?

  ....
  ....
  ....

- ## Record your weight: ....

Track Your Progress

Day ....   **Date**..................

- ## Diet Plan

  ....
  ....

- ## How do you feel?

  ....
  ....
  ....

- ## Record your weight: ....

Track Your Progress

Day ....   Date.................

- ## Diet Plan

  ....
  ....

- ## How do you feel?

  ....
  ....
  ....

- ## Record your weight: ....

Track Your Progress

Day ....   **Date**.................

- ### Diet Plan

  ....
  ....

- ### How do you feel?

  ....
  ....
  ....

- ### Record your weight: ....

KETO WORKBOOK
LIVE **& LOVE KETO**

<u>Track Your Progress</u>

Day ....   **Date**.................

- ## <u>Diet Plan</u>

> ....
>
> ....

- ## <u>How do you feel?</u>

> ....
>
> ....
>
> ....

- ## Record your weight: ....

Track Your Progress

Day ....   **Date**.................

- **Diet Plan**

- **How do you feel?**

- **Record your weight:** ....

<u>Track Your Progress</u>

Day ....   **Date**.................

- <u>**Diet Plan**</u>

> ....
>
> ....

- <u>**How do you feel?**</u>

> ....
>
> ....
>
> ....

- **Record your weight: ....**

LIVE

LOVE

KETO

Track Your Progress

Day ....   Date..................

- ### Diet Plan

....
....

- ### How do you feel?

....
....
....

- **Record your weight:** ....

<u>Track Your Progress</u>

Day ....   **Date**..................

- ## <u>Diet Plan</u>

....

....

- ## <u>How do you feel?</u>

....

....

....

- ## Record your weight: ....

Track Your Progress

Day ....   **Date**.................

- **Diet Plan**

  ....
  ....

- **How do you feel?**

  ....
  ....
  ....

- **Record your weight:** ....

Track Your Progress

Day ....   **Date**.................

- ## Diet Plan

  ....
  ....

- ## How do you feel?

  ....
  ....
  ....

- ## Record your weight: ....

Track Your Progress

Day .... Date.................

- ### Diet Plan

....
....

- ### How do you feel?

....
....

- **Record your weight: ....**

Track Your Progress

Day ....   **Date**.................

- ## Diet Plan

....
....

- ## How do you feel?

....
....

- **Record your weight:** ....

Track Your Progress

Day ....   **Date**.................

- **Diet Plan**

....
....
....

- **How do you feel?**

....
....
....
....

- **Record your weight:** ....

Track Your Progress

Day ....   **Date**................

- ## Diet Plan

....
....

- ## How do you feel?

....
....
....

- **Record your weight:** ....

Track Your Progress

Day ....   **Date**.................

- ## **Diet Plan**

  ....
  ....

- ## **How do you feel?**

  ....
  ....
  ....

- ## **Record your weight:** ....

Track Your Progress

Day ....   **Date**.................

- **Diet Plan**

  ....
  ....

- **How do you feel?**

  ....
  ....
  ....

- **Record your weight:** ....

Track Your Progress

Day ....   Date.................

- ### Diet Plan

  ....
  ....

- ## How do you feel?

  ....
  ....
  ....

- ## Record your weight: ....

Track Your Progress

Day .... Date..................

- ## Diet Plan

....
....

- ## How do you feel?

....
....
....

- **Record your weight: ....**

Track Your Progress

Day .... **Date**.................

- ## Diet Plan

....
....

- ## How do you feel?

....
....
....

- **Record your weight:** ....

Track Your Progress

Day .... Date.................

- ## Diet Plan

....
....
....

- ## How do you feel?

....
....
....
....

- ## Record your weight: ....

KEEP

LIVING

KETO